Contents

Chicken with cheese, prosciutto and roasted courgettes

Classic chicken Kiev with spring vegetables

Cumin and yoghurt chicken with cucumber and dill salad

Pulled chicken with barbecue sauce and baked potatoes

Kale and quinoa salad with orange tahini dressing

Peanut and dried mango-crusted partridge with curry leaf and tomato quinoa

Quinoa and halloumi burger

Cornish ling, grapefruit and prawn dressing, spiced quinoa and lemon yoghurt

Spiced monkfish tail with pickled beetroot and lemon, herby quinoa

BOTTOM LINE

development. Most people with multiple sclerosis are diagnosed between the ages of 20 and 40. Multiple sclerosis is rarely diagnosed in people under the age of 12 and over the age of 55.

The most definitive tool for diagnosing multiple sclerosis (MS) is magnetic resonance (MR) imaging and a new MR techni q ue called "Turbo FLAIR" in particular. There are no drugs or treatments which can cure multiple sclerosis, but treatments are now available which can modify the course of the disease. Life span is not significantly affected by multiple sclerosis, but the unpredictable physical and emotional effects of multiple sclerosis can be lifelong.

CHAPTER ONE

What is Multiple Sclerosis?

Multiple sclerosis (MS) is a neuroinflammatory disease that affects myelin , a substance that makes up the membrane (called the myelin sheath) that wraps around nerve fibers (axons). Myelinated axons are commonly called white matter. Researchers have learned that MS also damages the nerve cell bodies, which are found in the brain's gray matter, as well as the axons themselves in the brain, spinal cord, and optic nerve (the nerve that transmits visual information from the eye to the brain). As the disease progresses, the brain's cortex shrinks (cortical atrophy).

The term multiple sclerosis refers to the distinctive areas of scar tissue (sclerosis or plaques) that are visible in the white matter of people who have MS. Plaques can be as small as a pinhead or as large as the size of a golf ball. Doctors can see these areas by examining the brain and spinal cord using a type of brain scan called magnetic resonance imaging (MRI).

While MS sometimes causes severe disability, it is only rarely fatal and most people with MS have a normal life expectancy.

What are pla q ues made of and why do they develop?

Pla q ues, or lesions, are the result of an inflammatory process in the brain that causes immune system cells to attack myelin. The myelin sheath helps to speed nerve impulses traveling within the nervous system. Axons are also damaged in MS, although not as extensively, or as early in the disease, as myelin.

Under normal circumstances, cells of the immune system travel in and out of the brain patrolling for infectious agents (viruses, for example) or unhealthy cells. This is called the "surveillance" function of the immune system.

Surveillance cells usually won't spring into action unless they recognize an infectious agent or unhealthy cells. When they do, they produce substances to stop the infectious agent. If they encounter unhealthy cells, they either kill them directly or clean out the dying area and produce substances that promote healing and repair among the cells that are left.

Researchers have observed that immune cells behave differently in the brains of people with MS. They become active and attack what appears to be healthy myelin. It is unclear what triggers this attack. MS is one of many autoimmune disorders, such as rheumatoid arthritis and lupus, in which the immune system mistakenly attacks a person's healthy tissue as opposed to performing its normal role of attacking foreign invaders like viruses and bacteria. Whatever the reason, during these periods of immune system activity, most of the myelin within the affected area is damaged or destroyed. The axons also may be damaged. The symptoms of MS depend on the severity of the immune reaction as well as the location and extent of the pla q ues, which primarily appear in the brain stem, cerebellum, spinal cord, optic nerves, and the white matter of the brain around the brain ventricles (fluid-filled spaces inside of the brain).

What are the signs and symptoms of MS?

The symptoms of MS usually begin over one to several days, but in some forms, they may develop more slowly. They may be mild or severe and may go away q uickly or last for months. Sometimes the initial symptoms of MS are overlooked because they disappear in a day or so and normal function returns. Because symptoms come and go in the majority of people with MS, the presence of symptoms is called an attack, or in medical terms, an exacerbation. Recovery from symptoms is referred to as remission, while a return of symptoms is called a relapse. This form of MS is therefore called relapsing-remitting MS, in contrast to a more slowly developing form called primary progressive MS. Progressive MS can also be a second stage of the illness that follows years of relapsing-remitting symptoms.

A diagnosis of MS is often delayed because MS shares symptoms with other neurological conditions and diseases.

The first symptoms of MS often include:

vision problems such as blurred or double vision or optic neuritis, which causes pain in the eye and a rapid loss of vision

weak, stiff muscles, often with painful muscle spasms

tingling or numbness in the arms, legs, trunk of the body, or face

clumsiness, particularly difficulty staying balanced when walking

bladder control problems, either inability to control the bladder or urgency

dizziness that doesn't go away

MS may also cause later symptoms such as:

mental or physical fatigue which accompanies the above symptoms during an attack

mood changes such as depression or euphoria

changes in the ability to concentrate or to multitask effectively

difficulty making decisions, planning, or prioritizing at work or in private life.

Some people with MS develop transverse myelitis, a condition caused by inflammation in the spinal cord. Transverse myelitis causes loss of spinal cord function over a period of time lasting from several hours to several weeks. It usually begins as a sudden onset of lower back pain, muscle weakness, or abnormal sensations in the toes and feet, and can rapidly progress to more severe symptoms, including paralysis. In most cases of transverse myelitis, people recover at least some function within the first 12 weeks after an attack begins. Transverse myelitis can also result from viral infections, arteriovenous malformations, or neuroinflammatory problems unrelated to MS. In such instances, there are no pla q ues in the brain that suggest previous MS attacks.

Neuro-myelitis optica is a disorder associated with transverse myelitis as well as optic nerve inflammation. Patients with this disorder usually have antibodies against a particular protein in their spinal cord, called the a q uaporin channel. These patients respond differently to treatment than most people with MS.

Most individuals with MS have muscle weakness, often in their hands and legs. Muscle stiffness and spasms can also be a problem. These symptoms may be severe enough to affect walking or standing. In some cases, MS leads to partial or complete paralysis. Many people with MS find that weakness and fatigue are worse when they have a fever or when they are exposed to heat. MS exacerbations may occur following common infections.

Tingling and burning sensations are common, as well as the opposite, numbness and loss of sensation. Moving the neck from side to side or flexing it back and forth may cause "Lhermitte's sign," a characteristic sensation of MS that feels like a sharp spike of electricity coursing down the spine.

While it is rare for pain to be the first sign of MS, pain often occurs with optic neuritis and trigeminal neuralgia, a neurological disorder that affects one of the nerves that runs across the jaw, cheek, and face. Painful spasms of the limbs and sharp pain shooting down the legs or around the abdomen can also be symptoms of MS.

Most individuals with MS experience difficulties with coordination and balance at some time during the course of the disease. Some may have a continuous trembling of the head, limbs, and body, especially during movement, although such trembling is more common with other disorders such as Parkinson's disease.

Fatigue is common, especially during exacerbations of MS. A person with MS may be tired all the time or may be easily fatigued from mental or physical exertion.

Urinary symptoms, including loss of bladder control and sudden attacks of urgency, are common as MS progresses. People with MS sometimes also develop constipation or sexual problems.

Depression is a common feature of MS. A small number of individuals with MS may develop more severe psychiatric disorders such as bipolar disorder and paranoia, or experience inappropriate episodes of high spirits, known as euphoria.

People with MS, especially those who have had the disease for a long time, can experience difficulty with thinking, learning, memory, and judgment. The first signs of what doctors call cognitive dysfunction may be subtle. The person may have problems finding the right word to say, or trouble remembering how to do routine tasks on the job or at home. Day-to-day decisions that once came easily may now be made more slowly and show poor judgment. Changes may be so small or happen so slowly that it takes a family member or friend to point them out.

Types of MS

There are four types of MS:
Clinically isolated syndrome (CIS): This is a single, first episode, with symptoms lasting at least 24 hours. If another episode occurs at a later date, a doctor will diagnose relapse-remitting MS.

Relapse-remitting MS (RRMS): This is the most common form, affecting around 85% of people with MS. RRMS involves episodes of new or increasing symptoms, followed by periods of remission, during which symptoms go away partially or totally.

Primary progressive MS (PPMS): Symptoms worsen progressively, without early relapses or remissions. Some people may experience times of stability and periods when symptoms worsen and then get better. Around 15% of people with MS have PPMS.

Secondary progressive MS (SPMS): At first, people will experience episodes of relapse and remission, but then the disease will start to progress steadily.

Symptoms

Multiple sclerosis signs and symptoms may differ greatly from person to person and over the course of the disease depending on the location of affected nerve fibers. Symptoms often affect movement, such as:
• Numbness or weakness in one or more limbs that typically occurs on one side of your body at a time, or your legs and trunk
• Electric-shock sensations that occur with certain neck movements, especially bending the neck forward (Lhermitte sign)
• Tremor, lack of coordination or unsteady gait

Vision problems are also common, including:
• Partial or complete loss of vision, usually in one eye at a time, often with pain during eye movement
• Prolonged double vision
• Blurry vision

Multiple sclerosis symptoms may also include:
• Slurred speech

- Fatigue
- Dizziness
- Tingling or pain in parts of your body
- Problems with sexual, bowel and bladder function

When to see a doctor

See a doctor if you experience any of the above symptoms for unknown reasons.

Disease course

Most people with MS have a relapsing-remitting disease course. They experience periods of new symptoms or relapses that develop over days or weeks and usually improve partially or completely. These relapses are followed by quiet periods of disease remission that can last months or even years.

Small increases in body temperature can temporarily worsen signs and symptoms of MS, but these aren't considered true disease relapses.

At least 50% of those with relapsing-remitting MS eventually develop a steady progression of symptoms, with or without periods of remission, within 10 to 20 years from disease onset. This is known as secondary-progressive MS.

The worsening of symptoms usually includes problems with mobility and gait. The rate of disease progression varies greatly among people with secondary-progressive MS.

Some people with MS experience a gradual onset and steady progression of signs and symptoms without any relapses, known as primary-progressive MS.

Causes

The cause of multiple sclerosis is unknown. It's considered an autoimmune disease in which the body's immune system attacks its own tissues. In the case of MS, this immune system malfunction destroys the fatty substance that coats and protects nerve fibers in the brain and spinal cord (myelin).

Myelin can be compared to the insulation coating on electrical wires. When the protective myelin is damaged and the nerve fiber is exposed, the messages that travel along that nerve fiber may be slowed or blocked.

It isn't clear why MS develops in some people and not others. A combination of genetics and environmental factors appears to be responsible.

Risk factors

These factors may increase your risk of developing multiple sclerosis:
• Age. MS can occur at any age, but onset usually occurs around 20 and 40 years of age. However, younger and older people can be affected.
• Sex. Women are more than two to three times as likely as men are to have relapsing-remitting MS.
• Family history. If one of your parents or siblings has had MS, you are at higher risk of developing the disease.
• Certain infections. A variety of viruses have been linked to MS, including Epstein-Barr, the virus that causes infectious mononucleosis.
• Race. White people, particularly those of Northern European descent, are at highest risk of developing MS. People of Asian, African or Native American descent have the lowest risk.
• Climate. MS is far more common in countries with temperate climates, including Canada, the northern United States, New Zealand, southeastern Australia and Europe.
• Vitamin D. Having low levels of vitamin D and low exposure to sunlight is associated with a greater risk of MS.
• Certain autoimmune diseases. You have a slightly higher risk of developing MS if you have other autoimmune disorders such as thyroid disease, pernicious anemia, psoriasis, type 1 diabetes or inflammatory bowel disease.
• Smoking. Smokers who experience an initial event of symptoms that may signal MS are more likely than nonsmokers to develop a second event that confirms relapsing-remitting MS.

Complications

People with multiple sclerosis may also develop:
• Muscle stiffness or spasms
• Paralysis, typically in the legs
• Problems with bladder, bowel or sexual function
• Mental changes, such as forgetfulness or mood swings
• Depression

• Epilepsy

Diagnosis

There are no specific tests for MS. Instead, a diagnosis of multiple sclerosis often relies on ruling out other conditions that might produce similar signs and symptoms, known as a differential diagnosis.

Your doctor is likely to start with a thorough medical history and examination.

Your doctor may then recommend:

• Blood tests, to help rule out other diseases with symptoms similar to MS. Tests to check for specific biomarkers associated with MS are currently under development and may also aid in diagnosing the disease.

• Spinal tap (lumbar puncture), in which a small sample of cerebrospinal fluid is removed from your spinal canal for laboratory analysis. This sample can show abnormalities in antibodies that are associated with MS. A spinal tap can also help rule out infections and other conditions with symptoms similar to MS.

• MRI, which can reveal areas of MS (lesions) on your brain and spinal cord. You may receive an intravenous injection of a contrast material to highlight lesions that indicate your disease is in an active phase.

• Evoked potential tests, which record the electrical signals produced by your nervous system in response to stimuli. An evoked potential test may use visual stimuli or electrical stimuli. In these tests, you watch a moving visual pattern, or short electrical impulses are applied to nerves in your legs or arms. Electrodes measure how q uickly the information travels down your nerve pathways.

In most people with relapsing-remitting MS, the diagnosis is fairly straightforward and based on a pattern of symptoms consistent with the disease and confirmed by brain imaging scans, such as MRI.

Diagnosing MS can be more difficult in people with unusual symptoms or progressive disease. In these cases, further testing with spinal fluid analysis, evoked potentials and additional imaging may be needed.

Brain MRI is often used to help diagnose multiple sclerosis.

Treatment

There is no cure for multiple sclerosis. Treatment typically focuses on speeding recovery from attacks, slowing the progression of the disease and managing MS symptoms. Some people have such mild symptoms that no treatment is necessary.

Treatments for MS attacks

•   Corticosteroids, such as oral prednisone and intravenous methylprednisolone, are prescribed to reduce nerve inflammation. Side effects may include insomnia, increased blood pressure, increased blood glucose levels, mood swings and fluid retention.
• Plasma exchange (plasmapheresis). The liquid portion of part of your blood (plasma) is removed and separated from your blood cells. The blood cells are then mixed with a protein solution (albumin) and put back into your body. Plasma exchange may be used if your symptoms are new, severe and haven't responded to steroids.

Treatments to modify progression

For primary-progressive MS, ocrelizumab (Ocrevus) is the only FDA-approved disease-modifying therapy (DMT). Those who receive this treatment are slightly less likely to progress than those who are untreated.
For relapsing-remitting MS, several disease-modifying therapies are available.
Much of the immune response associated with MS occurs in the early stages of the disease. Aggressive treatment with these medications as early as possible can lower the relapse rate, slow the formation of new lesions, and potentially reduce risk of brain atrophy and disability accumulation.
Many of the disease-modifying therapies used to treat MS carry significant health risks. Selecting the right therapy for you will depend on careful consideration of many factors, including duration and severity of disease, effectiveness of previous MS treatments, other health issues, cost, and child-bearing status.
Treatment options for relapsing remitting MS include injectable and oral medications.
Injectable treatments include:

• Interferon beta medications.These drugs are among the most commonly prescribed medications to treat MS. They are injected under the skin or into muscle and can reduce the frequency and severity of relapses. Side effects of interferons may include flu-like symptoms and injection-site reactions. You'll need blood tests to monitor your liver enzymes because liver damage is a possible side effect of interferon use. People taking interferons may develop neutralizing antibodies that can reduce drug effectiveness.

• Glatiramer acetate (Copaxone, Glatopa). This medication may help block your immune system's attack on myelin and must be injected beneath the skin. Side effects may include skin irritation at the injection site.

Oral treatments include:

• Fingolimod (Gilenya). This once-daily oral medication reduces relapse rate. You'll need to have your heart rate and blood pressure monitored for six hours after the first dose because your heartbeat may be slowed. Other side effects include rare serious infections, headaches, high blood pressure and blurred vision.

• Dimethyl fumarate (Tecfidera). This twice-daily oral medication can reduce relapses. Side effects may include flushing, diarrhea, nausea and lowered white blood cell count. This drug requires blood test monitoring on a regular basis.

• Diroximel fumarate (Vumerity). This twice-daily capsule is similar to dimethyl fumarate but typically causes fewer side effects. It's approved for the treatment of relapsing forms of MS.

• Teriflunomide (Aubagio). This once-daily oral medication can reduce relapse rate. Teriflunomide can cause liver damage, hair loss and other side effects. This drug is associated with birth defects when taken by both men and women. Therefore, use contraception when taking this medication and for up to two years afterward. Couples who wish to become pregnant should talk to their doctor about ways to speed elimination of the drug from the body. This drug re q uires blood test monitoring in a regular basis.

• Siponimod (Mayzent). Research shows that this once-daily oral medication can reduce relapse rate and help slow progression of MS. It's also approved for secondary-progressive MS. Possible side effects include viral infections, liver problems and low white blood cell count. Other possible side effects include changes in heart rate, headaches and vision problems. Siponimod is harmful to a developing fetus, so women who may become pregnant should use contraception when taking this medication and for 10 days after stopping the medication. Some might need to have the heart rate and blood pressure monitored for six hours after the first dose. This drug re q uires blood test monitoring on a regular basis

• Cladribine (Mavenclad). This medication is generally prescribed as second line treatment for those with relapsing-remitting MS. It was also approved for secondary-progressive MS. It is given in two treatment courses, spread over a two-week period, over the course of two years. Side effects include upper respiratory infections, headaches, tumors, serious infections and reduced levels of white blood cells. People who have active chronic infections or cancer should not take this drug, nor should women who are pregnant or breast-feeding. Men and women should use contraception when taking this medication and for the following six months. You may need monitoring with blood tests while taking cladribine.

Infusion treatments include:

• Ocrelizumab (Ocrevus). This humanized monoclonal antibody medication is the only DMT approved by the FDA to treat both the relapse-remitting and primary-progressive forms of MS. Clinical trials showed that it reduced relapse rate in relapsing disease and slowed worsening of disability in both forms of the disease. Ocrelizumab is given via an intravenous infusion by a medical professional. Infusion-related side effects may include irritation at the injection site, low blood pressure, a fever and nausea, among others. Some people may not be able to take ocrelizumab, including those with a hepatitis B infection. Ocrelizumab may also increase the risk of infections and some types of cancer, particularly breast cancer.

• **Natalizumab (Tysabri).** This medication is designed to block the movement of potentially damaging immune cells from your bloodstream to your brain and spinal cord. It may be considered a first line treatment for some people with severe MS or as a second line treatment in others. This medication increases the risk of a potentially serious viral infection of the brain called progressive multifocal leukoencephalopathy (PML) in people who are positive for antibodies to the causative agent of PML JC virus. People who don't have the antibodies have extremely low risk of PML.

• **Alemtuzumab (Campath, Lemtrada).** This drug helps reduce relapses of MS by targeting a protein on the surface of immune cells and depleting white blood cells. This effect can limit potential nerve damage caused by the white blood cells. But it also increases the risk of infections and autoimmune disorders, including a high risk of thyroid autoimmune diseases and rare immune mediated kidney disease. Treatment with alemtuzumab involves five consecutive days of drug infusions followed by another three days of infusions a year later. Infusion reactions are common with alemtuzumab. The drug is only available from registered providers, and people treated with the drug must be registered in a special drug safety monitoring program. Alemtuzumab is usually recommended for those with aggressive MS or as second line treatment for patients who failed another MS medication.

Treatments for MS signs and symptoms

Physical therapy for multiple sclerosis
Physical therapy can build muscle strength and ease some of the symptoms of MS.

• **Physical therapy.** A physical or occupational therapist can teach you stretching and strengthening exercises and show you how to use devices to make it easier to perform daily tasks. Physical therapy along with the use of a mobility aid when necessary can also help manage leg weakness and other gait problems often associated with MS.

• **Muscle relaxants.** You may experience painful or uncontrollable muscle stiffness or spasms, particularly in your legs. Muscle relaxants such as baclofen (Lioresal, Gablofen), tizanidine (Zanaflex) and cyclobenzaprine may help. Onabotulinumtoxin A treatment is another option in those with spasticity.
• **Medications to reduce fatigue**. Amantadine (Gocovri, Osmolex), modafinil (Provigil) and methylphenidate (Ritalin) may be helpful in reducing MS-related fatigue. Some drugs used to treat depression, including selective serotonin reuptake inhibitors, may be recommended.

• **Medication to increase walking speed.** Dalfampridine (Ampyra) may help to slightly increase walking speed in some people. People with a history of seizures or kidney dysfunction should not take this medication.
• Other medications. Medications also may be prescribed for depression, pain, sexual dysfunction, insomnia, and bladder or bowel control problems that are associated with MS.

Lifestyle and home remedies

To help relieve the signs and symptoms of MS, try to:
• **Get plenty of rest.** Look at your sleep habits to make sure you're getting the best possible sleep. To make sure you're getting enough sleep, you may need to be evaluated — and possibly treated — for sleep disorders such as obstructive sleep apnea.

• **Exercise.** If you have mild to moderate MS, regular exercise can help improve your strength, muscle tone, balance and coordination. Swimming or other water exercises are good options if you're bothered by heat. Other types of mild to moderate exercise recommended for people with MS include walking, stretching, low-impact aerobics, stationary bicycling, yoga and tai chi.

• **Cool down.** MS symptoms often worsen when the body temperature rises in some people with MS. Avoiding exposure to heat and using devices such as cooling scarves or vests can be helpful.

• **Eat a balanced diet.** Since there's little evidence to support a particular diet, experts recommend a generally healthy diet. Some research suggests that vitamin D may have potential benefit for people with MS.

• **Relieve stress.** Stress may trigger or worsen your signs and symptoms. Yoga, tai chi, massage, meditation or deep breathing may help.

Alternative medicine

Many people with MS use a variety of alternative or complementary treatments or both to help manage their symptoms, such as fatigue and muscle pain.

Activities such as exercise, meditation, yoga, massage, eating a healthier diet, acupuncture and relaxation techniques may help boost overall mental and physical well-being, but there are few studies to back up their use in managing symptoms of MS.

According to guidelines from the American Academy of Neurology, research strongly indicates that oral cannabis extract (OCE) may improve symptoms of muscle spasticity and pain. There is a lack of evidence that cannabis in any other form is effective in managing other MS symptoms.

Daily intake of vitamin D3 of 2,000-5,000 international units daily is recommended in those with MS. The connection between vitamin D and MS is supported by the association with exposure to sunlight and the risk of MS.

How does diet affect MS?

Currently, there are no official dietary guidelines for people with MS. No two people with MS experience it the same way.

However, scientists believe a combination of genetic and environmental factors may cause the disease, as well as that nutrition can have an influence. The fact that MS is more prevalent in Western countries than in developing nations is one clue that diet may play a key role.

That is why dietary guidelines and recommendations for people with MS should aim to help manage symptoms to improve overall q uality of life.

Diet may help with MS in several ways, including by preventing or controlling its progression, helping manage its symptoms, and reducing flare-ups.

Ideally, an MS-friendly diet should be high in antioxidants to fight inflammation, high in fiber to aid bowel movements, ade q uate in calcium and vitamin D to fight osteoporosis, and pack plenty of vitamins and minerals to fight fatigue and promote wellness.

It should also limit foods that have been linked to chronic inflammation and other poor health outcomes, or those that simply make day-to-day activities more difficult for someone with MS.

Some evidence suggests that other dietary patterns, including ketogenic diets, may help improve symptoms in people with MS. However, this research is ongoing, and scientists need to further investigate the role of diet in MS.

A study in 60 people with MS found that fast-mimicking diets and ketogenic diets had potential to treat relapsing-remitting multiple sclerosis (RRMS). Still, the researchers suggested that more high quality studies on the effects of fast-mimicking diets in humans were needed.

Another study that gave people with MS a ketogenic diet found they showed improved symptoms, including reduced fatigue, inflammation, and depression.

A separate study found certain nutrients may benefit people with mild to moderate MS, potentially leading to better general functioning, as well as an improved q uality of life and ability to move around.

The nutrients associated with these positive changes included increased fat, cholesterol, folate, iron, and magnesium intakes. On the other hand, decreased carb intake appeared to be beneficial.

Clinical trials investigating the effects of ketogenic diets and intermittent fasting on MS are currently underway.

Current evidence suggests that a modified paleolithic diet and taking supplements may help improve perceived fatigue in MS patients.

There's also evidence that people with MS are more likely to be deficient in some nutrients, including vitamins A, B12, and D3.

Preliminary evidence suggests that taking certain vitamins, minerals, fatty acids, antioxidants, plant compounds, and melatonin may help improve some symptoms.

Scientists need to do more research before making official recommendations about many of the dietary patterns discussed above. However, preliminary research is promising.

Foods to eat

Certain foods may benefit people with MS by affecting how the immune system, the nerves, and other parts of the body work.

Probiotics and prebiotics

Changes in gut health may contribute to immune disorders, and research indicates that the health of the gut appears to play a role in many kinds of diseases.

The intestinal flora, or gut flora, is a highly complex system of microorganisms that live in the intestines. In humans, these microorganisms are largely bacteria.

The bacteria are responsible for breaking down food and nutrients, and they play a key role in digestion and the health of the immune system. Healthy gut flora thrive in the intestines when there is ample fiber in the diet.

A lack of healthy gut flora may contribute to a range of immune disorders, including MS. Anyone with the condition should have a diet that supports a healthy immune system, and one that promotes beneficial gut flora may help.

Probiotics are foods that can boost levels of beneficial bacteria in the gut, helping to strengthen the immune system.

The authors of a study in Nature Communications suggest that adjusting the gut flora, by using probiotics, for example, may be helpful for people with MS.

Probiotic bacteria are available in supplements and a range of fermented foods. The following all contain healthful levels of Lactobacillus, which is one type of beneficial bacteria:

• Yogurt
• Kefir
• Kimchi
• Sauerkraut
• Kombucha, or fermented tea

Prebiotics

After filling the gut with good bacteria, it is important to feed them. Foods that nourish probiotic bacteria are called prebiotics, and they contain fiber.

Foods that contain healthful levels of prebiotic fiber include:

• Artichokes
• Garlic
• Leeks
• Asparagus
• Onions
• Chicory

Fiber

Fiber occurs in plant-based foods, such as:

• Fruits
• Vegetables
• Nuts and seeds
• Legumes, such as lentils
• Whole grains
• Brown rice

It helps promote health in the following ways:

• nourishing the gut bacteria
• encouraging regular bowel movements
• keeping blood pressure and the heart healthy by helping manage cholesterol
• reducing the risk of weight gain by leaving a person feeling full for longer
People with MS may have a higher risk of certain types of heart disease. While dietary measures may not reduce these risks, a healthful diet will benefit overall heart health.

Vitamin D

Vitamin D is important for everyone, but it may be especially beneficial for people with MS. According to the National Institute of Neurological Disorders and Stroke, people with high levels of vitamin D appear to have a lower chance of developing MS.

Vitamin D is also important for bone health. People with MS may be more likely to experience low bone density and osteoporosis, especially if they are not able to move easily. An ade q uate intake of vitamin D may help prevent this.

Most of the body's vitamin D comes from exposure to sunlight, but a person also takes it in by consuming:
• Oily fish
• Fortified dairy products
• Some fortified cereals, yogurt, and orange juice
• Beef liver
• Egg yolks

A review published in 2017 notes that, while evidence of a link between low vitamin D levels and MS is accumulating, confirming the link will require more research.

Biotin

Biotin is a form of vitamin B, and some people call it vitamin H.
It occurs in many foods, but good sources include:
• Eggs
• Yeast
• Beef liver

• Sunflower seeds
• Almonds
• Spinach
• Broccoli
• Whole-wheat bread

Researchers have been looking into whether biotin might benefit people with MS. Findings from small studies indicate that a high dosage of biotin — between 100 and 600 milligrams per day — could help people with progressive MS, in which symptoms gradually become more severe.

Confirming and specifying the benefits of biotin supplementation will re q uire more research, but following a healthful diet can often ensure that a person is consuming enough of this vitamin.

Polyunsaturated fatty acids

Investigations into whether a diet rich in polyunsaturated fatty acids (PUFAs) directly helps relieve MS symptoms have yielded mixed results. However, there is evidence that these acids help support a healthy body and control inflammation.

A study published in 2017 concluded that a low intake of PUFAs may increase the risk of MS. The study looked at data from more than 170,000 women.

PUFAs appear to boost bodily functions ranging from cardiac health to the ability to think. Examples of foods that contain PUFAs include fatty fish, such as salmon and mackerel, and some plant-based oils.

Antioxidants

Many vegetable-based foods contain substances called polyphenols, which have antioxidantand anti-inflammatory effects on the body's cells. These effects may help prevent cell damage, making polyphenols potentially useful for people with MS.

Sources of polyphenols include:
• Fruits
• Vegetables
• Spices
• Cereals
• Legumes
• Fruits

• Herbs
• Tea
Antioxidants can also help prevent oxidative stress, which researchers have linked to a wide range of health problems.
Some antioxidants — specifically resveratrol, which occurs in grapes — appear to help protect the nervous system.
Weight management
A review published in 2016 concluded that obesity during childhood and adolescence might increase the risk of developing MS. The researchers also noted that obesity could affect the progression of the disease.
In addition, a person with MS who loses mobility or who finds movement more challenging may have a higher risk of putting on extra weight.
Managing the diet to prevent weight gain may also help prevent MS symptoms from worsening. These types of dietary changes may boost a person's sense of well-being and reduce the risk of additional health conditions, such as cardiovascular disease.
For more science-backed resources on nutrition, visit our dedicated hub.

Foods to avoid

Some foods may be harmful to people with MS.
Saturated fats and processed foods
Processed foods can have a negative impact on a person's health, especially if they contain high levels of:
• saturated fats, Trans fats, and hydrogenated oils
• Added sodium, or salt
• Added sugar
Sodium
A article published in ASN Neuro in 2015 noted that people with MS who have a moderate or high sodium intake are more likely to experience a relapse of symptoms or develop a new lesion.

The authors also suggested avoiding:
• Sugar-sweetened drinks
• Excessive q uantities of red meat
• Fried foods
• Low-fiber foods

These, they point out, can trigger inflammation in the body. A healthful diet that includes fresh fruits and vegetables can reduce inflammation, due to its antioxidant effects.

Special diets: Can they help with MS?

Anyone on a specific diet needs to be sure that they are consuming all the required daily nutrients. A person who eliminates a particular food or food group should ensure that they replace any nutrients lost.

Gluten-free diet

Research has not confirmed a link between gluten and MS, but people with MS appear to have a higher likelihood of developing celiac disease, which prevents the body from tolerating gluten. Both diseases seem to stem from a problem with the immune system.

Foods that contain gluten include:

• wheat products, such as breads, baked goods, and many premade soups and salad dressings
• barley products, such as malt, soups, beer, and brewer's yeast
• Rye, which is often present in bread, rye beer, and cereals

People who follow a gluten-free diet may miss out on important nutrients, including fiber, which is present in whole grains. They should boost their fiber intake by eating plenty of fresh vegetables, fruits, nuts, seeds, and pulses.

Anyone considering a gluten-free diet should speak to their doctor first.

Paleo diet

Many people on the Paleo, or Paleolithic, diet believe that the human body has not evolved to eat the highly processed foods that we now consume.

The diet involves switching to foods that were likely eaten by hunter-gatherers. The first step is to choose natural foods over processed foods, with an emphasis on meat and plant-based foods, but not grains.

In a 2019 review, researchers, including an advocate of the Paleo diet, compared a modified version of it with another diet — the Swank diet — to test, among other factors, the effects on MS-related fatigue. There is some evidence that the diets may reduce this fatigue, but confirming this will require more research.

Swank diet

Doctors developed the Swank diet as an MS treatment in the 1950s. It reduces saturated fat intake to, at most, 15 grams per day and recommends limiting unsaturated fat intake to 20–50 grams per day.

People on this diet:
• Cannot eat processed foods or dairy fats
• Cannot eat red meat, during the first year
• Can eat as much white fish and shellfish as they like
• should eat at least 2 cups each of fruits and vegetables every day
• should eat whole-grain pasta
• should take cod liver oil and multivitamins every day
While some consider the diet to be dated, others report that it helps.
Possible risks include deficiencies in folic acid and vitamins A, C, and E.

How do the diets compare?

In 2015, the National MS Society reviewed a number of diets and their impact on the disease. The authors conclude that there is not enough evidence to recommend one diet over another and acknowledge that most of the diets restrict or leave out the same types of food.

A person should avoid foods that:
• Are highly processed
• Are high in saturated fat
• have high glycemic index ratings, suggesting that they contain high levels of sugar or are significantly processed

In general, the diets tend to involve eating:
• Less fatty red meat
• More fruits and vegetables

CHAPTER TWO

<u>Recipes to try while on a multiple sclerosis diet</u>

Salmon coulibiac with roasted vegetables

Ingredients
For the salmon coulibiac
• 900g/2lb readymade all-butter puff pastry
• 1.2kg/2lb 12oz whole salmon fillet
• 300ml/7fl oz double cream
• 5 tbsp chives, finely chopped
• 500g/1lb 2oz spinach, blanched in boiling water for one minute, refreshed in cold water and squeezed dry
• 1 free-range egg, beaten
For the roasted vegetables
• 2 red onions, peeled and cut into wedges
• 3 large carrots, peeled and cut into chunks
• 3 large parsnips, peeled and cut into chunks
• 3 tbsp olive oil

For the beurre blanc
• 2 shallots, peeled, finely sliced
• 1 tbsp white wine vinegar
• 4 tbsp white wine
• 225g/8oz butter, cut into cubes
• Salt and freshly ground black pepper
• 4 tbsp chopped chives

Method
1. Preheat the oven to 210C/425F/Gas7. Line a baking tray with silicone or baking parchment.
2. For the salmon coulibiac, roll the pastry out to a thickness of 5mm and cut into two pieces about 40 x 25cm /16 x 10in. Place one piece onto the lined baking tray.
3. Cut off 2/3 of the whole fillet (roughly 800g), place on top of the pastry on

the tray in the centre then cover with half the blanched spinach.

4. Roughly chop the remaining salmon (about 400g) and place into a food processor with the double cream and half the chives. Blend to a purée.

5. Season with salt and plenty of freshly ground black pepper, then spread over the top of the spinach to cover completely.

6. Finish with a scattering of chives and the rest of the spinach. Brush the pastry around the fish with a little of the beaten egg.

7. Lay the second piece of pastry over the top, taking care not to stretch it and press down firmly around the edge of the salmon.

8. Trim the edges with a sharp knife so there is only a little overlap around the edge. Brush the coulibiac all over with egg and season with salt and black pepper.

9. Place onto a baking tray in the oven and bake for 40-45 minutes until the salmon is cooked through and the pastry golden-brown.

10. For the roasted vegetables, place all the ingredients onto a roasting tray tossing the vegetables to coat with the olive oil. Season with salt and black pepper. Roast for 25-35 minutes until tender.

11. For the beurre blanc, bring the finely sliced shallots, white wine vinegar and white wine to the boil in a saucepan. Reduce the heat until the mixture is simmering, then continue to simmer until only two tablespoons of liquid are left in the pan.

12. Add one tablespoon of cold water and continue to simmer until only one tablespoon of li q uid remains.

13. Reduce the heat to low, then gradually whisk in the butter, 25g/1oz at a time, waiting until all of the butter has melted and incorporated into the mixture before adding more.

14. Remove the mixture from the heat and strain it into a clean saucepan. Season, to taste, with salt and freshly ground black pepper, then stir in the chives. Set aside at room temperature until needed (do not refrigerate as the sauce will separate).

15. To serve, carve the salmon into thick slices and place onto a plate.

16. Pile the vegetables alongside and finish with a drizzle of beurre blanc.

Salmon in pastry with dill and ginger

Ingredients
• 150g/5½oz softened unsalted butter

- pinch mace
- 1 bunch fresh dill, chopped
- 100g/3½oz currants
- 4-6 pieces stem ginger, finely chopped
- Salt and pepper, to taste
- 2 thick pieces salmon, about 600g/1lb 5oz each filleted, pin-boned and skinned
- 1kg/2lb 4oz puff pastry
- 1 free-range egg, beaten

For the butter sauce
- 2 tbsp white wine vinegar
- 150ml/5fl oz white wine
- 1 banana shallot, chopped
- 250g/9oz unsalted butter

Method
1. Preheat the oven to 190C/170C Fan/Gas 5 and line a baking tray with parchment.
2. Mix together the butter, mace, dill, currants, ginger, salt and pepper in a bowl to make a paste. Place one piece of salmon on a clean work surface, smear the paste on top and lay the other fillet on top of the paste.
3. Cut the pastry in half and roll out each piece to about 2cm/¾ wider than the size of the salmon. Place one piece of pastry on the lined baking tray and lay the salmon on top. Dab water around the edge of the pastry, then lay the other piece of pastry on top. Press the edges together lightly to seal.
4. Glaze the top of the parcel with the beaten egg and crimp the edges to finish. Chill in the fridge for 20 minutes and then brush with egg again. Bake for 30 minutes, or until golden-brown.
5. For the butter sauce place the vinegar, white wine and shallots into a saucepan and cook until reduced in volume by half. Gradually whisk in the butter until a smooth sauce is formed. Season with salt and pepper.
6. Cut the salmon into slices and serve with the butter sauce.

Prawn and salmon terrine with dill sauce

Ingredients

- 200g/7oz salmon
- 350–400g/12–14oz smoked salmon, preferably in long strips
- 150g/5½oz cooked prawns
- 1 lime, finely grated zest and juice
- 100ml/3½fl oz double cream
- 100ml/3½fl oz single cream
- 4 leaves gelatine, soaked in cold water
- Few fresh sprigs dill, finely chopped
- Few fresh chives, finely snipped
- salt and freshly ground black pepper

For the dill sauce
- ½ cucumber, seeds removed, coarsely grated or thinly sliced
- 300ml/10fl oz plain yoghurt or soured cream
- 2 tsp cider vinegar
- ½ lime, juice only
- small bunch fresh dill

Method

1. Preheat the oven to 200C/180C Fan/Gas 6. Wrap the salmon in foil and put it on a baking tray. Bake for 12–15 minutes, or until just cooked.

2. Meanwhile, line a narrow 450g/1lb loaf tin with cling film, making sure plenty is overhanging. Line the sides of the tin with the smoked salmon – the easiest way to do this is across, making sure you leave enough hanging over the sides to cover the top.

3. Flake the cooked salmon and finely chop the cooked prawns. Put them in a bowl and add the lime juice and zest. Season with salt and pepper.

4. In a second bowl, lightly whip the double cream until it is just approaching the stage when soft peaks form when the whisk is removed from the bowl.

5. Heat the single cream in a saucepan. Squeeze out the gelatine when it is soft and add it to the single cream. Stir until the gelatine has dissolved.

6. Fold the double cream through the prawns and salmon, then pour in the single cream and gelatine mixture, preferably through a sieve. Add the herbs and mix well. Season if necessary.

7. Spoon the mixture into the smoked salmon-lined terrine and smooth over. Fold over the overhanging pieces of smoked salmon followed by the cling film. Transfer to the fridge and leave for several hours to set and chill.

8. To make the dill sauce, sprinkle the cucumber with salt and leave to stand

for 30 minutes in a colander – this will help get rid of some of the excess li q uid. S q ueeze out the water.

9. Put the yoghurt in a bowl and add the vinegar and lime juice. Stir in the cucumber and dill, then taste. Cover and chill in the fridge.

10. Remove the terrine from the dish and peel off the cling film. Slice the terrine and serve on a plate with the dill sauce.

Salmon enpapillote with herb salad

Ingredients
For the salmon
• 1 red onion, thinly sliced
• 1 large carrot, peeled and julienned
• 2 garlic cloves, grated
• 30g/1oz fresh root ginger, peeled and julienned
• 50g/1¾oz mangetout, julienned
• 1 red chilli, seeds removed and julienned
• 1 tsp mild curry powder
• 2 spring onions, trimmed and thinly sliced
• 200ml/7fl oz coconut milk
• 100ml/3½fl oz white wine
• 2 x 150g/5½oz centre-cut salmon fillets, skin on
• 16 large mussels, scrubbed and debearded
• 30g/1oz crème fraîche
• 1 lime, juice only
• Salt and freshly ground black pepper

For the herb salad
• 2 tbsp chopped fresh dill
• 2 tbsp chopped fresh chervil
• 2 tbsp chopped fresh coriander
• 2 tbsp chopped fresh pea shoots
• 2 tbsp olive oil

Method
1. Preheat the oven to 220C/200C Fan/Gas 7.
2. To make the salmon, mix the red onion, carrot, garlic, ginger, mangetout,

chili, curry powder and spring onion in a bowl and season with salt and pepper. Mix the coconut milk and wine in a separate bowl and set aside.

3. Cut out four large s q uares of kitchen foil and baking paper. Place the foil squares on top of the baking paper squares in order to start making two parcel shapes. Place the salmon pieces on one half of each parcel s q uare. Place the vegetables on top of the salmon and place the mussels around the fish. Discard any mussels with broken shells and any that refuse to close when tapped.

4. Fold the free half of each parcel s q uare over the salmon and fold up all the edges to create parcels, sealing at every fold until you reach the last corners. Pour in the wine mixture and then seal each parcel tightly. Cook in the preheated oven for 9 minutes, or until the salmon is cooked through, then take out and rest for 1 minute. Remove the fish and mussels from the parcels, remove the salmon skin and keep warm. Discard any mussels that remain closed.

5. To make the herb salad, place the herbs in a large bowl. Transfer the vegetables from the parcels to the bowl and stir in the olive oil.

6. Add the juices from the parcels to a saucepan and bring to the boil. Add the crème fraîche and whisk. Stir in the lime juice.

7. Serve the herb salad on top of the fish and mussels and pour over the sauce.

Couscous-coated goujons of salmon with warm tomato and herb salsa

Ingredients

For the salmon goujons
- Vegetable oil, for deep frying
- 100g/3½oz salmon fillet, skin removed
- 1 free-range egg, beaten
- 55g/2oz couscous

For the tomato salsa
- 1 tbsp olive oil
- 1 garlic clove, finely chopped
- 2 tomatoes, chopped
- ¼ tsp dried chilli flakes

- 1 tbsp balsamic vinegar
- Chopped fresh parsley, to garnish

Method

1. For the salmon goujons, place the vegetable oil into a deep, heavy-based saucepan and heat until a small cube of bread sizzles and turns golden when dropped into it. (CAUTION: hot oil can be dangerous. Do not leave unattended.)

2. Slice the salmon into four long strips. Dip the salmon strips in the beaten egg.

3. Sprinkle the couscous onto a plate and coat the salmon slices in the couscous.

4. Carefully place the salmon into the hot oil and deep fry for about 3-4 minutes, or until crisp and cooked through. Remove from the oil with a slotted spoon and drain on kitchen paper.

5. For the tomato salsa, heat the oil in a frying pan. Add the garlic, tomatoes and chilli flakes and simmer for 2-3 minutes. Stir in the balsamic vinegar.

6. Serve the salmon goujons on a plate with the salsa and garnish with parsley.

Poached salmon with asparagus

Ingredients
- 1kg/2lb 4oz side of salmon
- Small bunch dill
- 50ml/2fl oz dry white wine
- 1 lemon, juice only
- Salt and freshly ground black pepper

For the garnish
- 20 asparagus tips
- 100g/3½oz cooked shelled brown shrimps
- Pink radishes or pink micro herbs

For the dressing
- ½ banana shallot, finely diced
- 2 tsp Dijon mustard

- 3 tbsp white wine vinegar
- 150ml/5fl oz light olive oil
- 1 tsp caster sugar
- Bunch fresh dill, chopped

Method
1. Preheat the oven to 180C/160C Fan/Gas 4.
2. Lightly butter a large sheet of kitchen foil big enough to wrap the salmon.
3. Put a few sprigs of dill to one side of the foil. Season the foil and place the salmon on top, skin-side up. Pour over the white wine and lemon juice. Fold the foil over the fish to make a parcel, sealing the edges at the side.
4. Lift into a large roasting tin and bake for about 25 minutes, or until just cooked, pale pink and matte. Leave to rest for 10 minutes, then carefully remove the skin and scrape off any grey fat.
5. To make the garnish, blanch the asparagus in a pan of boiling water for 3 minutes. Drain and refresh under cold water. Cut into small pieces.
6. To make the dressing, mix all of the dressing ingredients together in a jug.
7. Using two fish slices, transfer the salmon onto a serving platter. Arrange the asparagus along the length of the fish, scatter the shrimps over the top and spoon over some of the dressing. Garnish with slices of radish or micro herbs.
8. Serve with the remaining dressing in a jug.

Seared salmon with asparagus salsa

Ingredients
For the salmon
- 1 lemon, zest only
- 1 lime, zest only
- 2 tbsp coarse sea salt
- 320g/11oz fresh salmon fillet, skin removed, cut in half lengthways
- 1 tbsp smoked paprika
- 1 tbsp olive oil

For the asparagus salsa
- 1 bunch English asparagus, woody ends removed
- ½ red chilli, seeds removed, cut into small thin strips

- ½ red onion, finely chopped
- ½ cucumber, peeled and seeds removed, cut into 1cm/½in cubes
- 3 heirloom tomatoes, skinned and seeds removed, cut into 1cm/½in cubes
- ½ lime, peeled, pith removed, finely chopped
- 2 tbsp white balsamic vinegar
- few drops Tabasco sauce
- salt and freshly ground black pepper
- 1 tbsp chopped fresh coriander

Method

1. For the salmon, mix the lemon and lime zests with the salt in a small bowl, then rub the mixture onto the salmon. Cover with clingfilm and marinate in the fridge for 15 minutes.

2. Brush the salt mixture off the salmon and pat dry.

3. Heat a frying pan or griddle over a high heat. Drizzle the olive oil over the salmon fillets and fry for 30 seconds on each side. Remove the salmon from the frying pan, dust with paprika, wrap in clingfilm and set aside to cool.

4. For the asparagus salsa, reserve 5cm/2in of the tips and slice the remaining stems into thin rounds. Slice the tips thinly using a Japanese slicer or vegetable peeler and set aside.

5. Mix the asparagus stems, chilli, red onion, cucumber, tomatoes and lime together in a bowl. Add the balsamic vinegar and a few drops of Tabasco sauce, to taste. Season with salt and freshly ground black pepper.

6. To serve, spoon the salsa onto serving plates. Slice the salmon into eight slices and add two slices to each serving plate. Sprinkle over the coriander and top with the asparagus tips.

Salmon confit with crushed new potatoes

Ingredients

For the salmon confit

- 500ml/18fl oz olive oil
- 1 garlic clove, finely chopped
- 4 x 140g/5oz salmon fillets, skin on (or mackerel, sardines or any smoked fish)
- Bunch fresh coriander, chopped, to serve
- 2 Little Gem lettuces, chopped, to serve (or any other salad or green leaves)

For the crushed potatoes
• 600g/1lb 5oz new potatoes, such as Jersey Royal potatoes, scrubbed
• 1 tbsp snipped fresh chives
• 2 tsp chopped fresh dill
• 25g/1oz butter
• salt and freshly ground black pepper

For the dressing
• 1 tbsp chopped fresh dill
• 4 tbsp extra virgin olive oil
• ½ lime (or lemon), juice only

Method
1. To make the salmon confit, pour the olive oil into a large heavy-based saucepan or casserole that will fit the salmon fillets snugly. Add the garlic and gently heat the oil for a few minutes to let the flavours infuse. Add the salmon fillets to the pan. Cook over a low heat for 8 minutes (or 10 minutes if you prefer your fish well cooked), then take off the heat. Leave the salmon in the oil for 5 minutes, then transfer to kitchen paper to drain.
2. Meanwhile, to make the crushed potatoes, put the potatoes into a saucepan of boiling water and simmer for 15 minutes or until tender. Drain, place the potatoes into a large bowl and lightly crush with a fork. Add the chives, dill, butter and a drizzle of oil from the salmon. Season with salt and pepper and mix well.
3. To make the dressing, whisk the dill, olive oil and lime juice together in a jug or small bowl.
4. To serve, place cooking rings on six plates and fill each ring with the crushed potatoes (if you don't have a ring, spoon into a neat pile instead). Remove the ring and lay a salmon fillet next to the potatoes. Mix the coriander and lettuce together and serve a small amount on each plate. Spoon over the dressing and serve.

Crisp roasted salmon with sweet and sour peppers

Ingredients
For the roasted salmon
• 1 tsp olive oil

• 125g/4½oz salmon fillet, skin on
• salt and freshly ground black pepper

For the sweet and sour peppers
• 1 tbsp olive oil
• 1 red pepper, seeds removed, chopped
• 1 yellow pepper, seeds removed, chopped
• 2 tbsp red wine vinegar
• Pinch caster sugar

To serve
• Handful mixed salad leaves
• Balsamic vinegar, for drizzling

Method
1. Preheat the oven to 180C/350F/Gas 4.
2. For the roasted salmon, rub the olive oil into the salmon and season well with salt and freshly ground black pepper.
3. Heat an ovenproof frying pan over a high heat. Add the salmon, skin-side down first, and fry for 1-2 minutes, or until the skin is crisp. Turn the salmon over and fry for 30 seconds to one minute to sear the fish. Turn it over again so it is laying skin-side down and transfer the pan to the oven for 7-8 minutes to roast the salmon.
4. For the sweet and sour peppers, heat the oil in a separate non-reactive frying pan over a medium heat. Add the pepper pieces and fry for 2-3 minutes, or until they start to soften.
5. Add the red wine vinegar and sugar and continue to cook for 5-6 minutes, or until the peppers are soft and the vinegar has reduced.
6. To serve, scatter the mixed leaves onto a serving plate, and place the crisp roasted salmon on top. Arrange the peppers around the edge of the plate. Drizzle the dish with balsamic vinegar.

Griddled asparagus with pan-fried salmon and olive paste

Ingredients
For the olive paste
• 150g/5oz black olives, pitted

- 1 tbsp chives
- 1 tbsp fresh coriander leaves
- 3 tbsp olive oil
- Handful fresh basil leaves

For the asparagus
- Drizzle olive oil
- 4 asparagus spears, blanched in boiling water
- Salt and freshly ground black pepper

For the salmon
- 150g/5oz salmon fillet

Method
1. Preheat the oven to 220C/425F/Gas 7.
2. To make the olive paste, place the olives, chives, coriander, olive oil and basil into a food processor and blend until smooth.
3. Meanwhile, for the asparagus, heat the oil in an ovenproof griddle pan until smoking. Add the asparagus spears and chargrill for 2-3 minutes. Season, to taste, with salt and freshly ground black pepper. Remove from the pan and keep warm.
4. For the salmon, place the salmon fillet onto the hot griddle pan and cook for 1-2 minutes, until browned. Turn over the salmon and spread with the olive paste. Transfer the salmon to the oven and to roast for a 5-6 minutes, until the salmon is completely cooked through.
5. To serve, arrange the griddled asparagus spears on a plate and top with the salmon.

Ras-el-hanout chicken wraps with a yoghurt sauce

Ingredients
For the ras-el-hanout chicken wraps
- 4 large chicken breasts
- 2 heaped tbsp ras-el-hanout spice mix

- 7-8 tbsp olive oil
- Sea salt, to taste
- 2-3 tbsp pomegranate molasses, to taste
- Rocket or lettuce leaves, to serve
- 4-6 flour tortillas

For the yoghurt sauce
- 400g/14oz full-fat Greek yoghurt
- 1 small bunch fresh mint, finely chopped
- 2 tbsp sumac
- sea salt and freshly ground black pepper

Method

1. For the ras-el-hanout chicken wraps, cut the thick side of each chicken breast horizontally to even out the thickness of each breast and ensure they cook evenly. In a small bowl, mix the ras-el-hanout with 4-5 tablespoons of the olive oil to create a paste. Smear the paste over the chicken breasts, ensuring they are well coated. Season each breast with a pinch of sea salt, cover with cling film and place in the fridge to marinate for at least 10 minutes and up to a few hours.

2. To make the yoghurt sauce, put the yoghurt, fresh mint and sumac in a small serving bowl. Season with a generous pinch of sea salt and some black pepper. Mix well until the sumac and mint are evenly incorporated.

3. For the ras-el-hanout chicken wraps, preheat a large frying pan over a medium heat. Add the remaining olive oil and the chicken breasts (you may want to use two pans at a time if cooking all four chicken breasts at once). Fry the chicken for about 8-10 minutes on one side and 6-8 minutes on the other side. You can check how cooked the chicken is by prodding the fattest part of the chicken strips with your finger - if it feels very springy then it needs to cook a bit longer. Check the chicken is cooked by piercing the thickest part with a skewer or small knife. If the juices run clear and the flesh is no longer pink then the chicken is cooked and ready to serve. Place your cooked chicken on a chopping board and allow to rest for a few minutes before slicing into strips.

4. To serve, put a few strips of chicken on each tortilla wrap, add a dollop of the yoghurt sauce and then drizzle with pomegranate molasses. Add some rocket or lettuce leaves, roll up the tortillas and serve.

Tex-Mex brick chicken

Ingredients
For the chicken
- 2 dried chipotle chillies
- ¼-½ habanero chilli, to taste
- Generous pinch sea salt flakes
- 4 tbsp olive oil
- 1 orange, juice only
- 2 tsp fresh oregano leaves
- 2 garlic cloves, roughly chopped
- 1 large whole chicken, spatchcocked and de-boned, only wing bones left in (ask your butcher to do this for you)

For the frijoles
- Large knob of butter
- 1 onion, finely chopped
- 2 garlic cloves, finely chopped
- ½ bunch fresh coriander, stalks chopped, leaves reserved for garnish
- 2 x 400g tins good- q uality Mexican black beans
- 1 small red chilli, finely chopped, to garnish

To serve
- 4-8 soft tacos
- Handful grated Mexican-style firm cheese, such as Oaxaca (available from specialist cheese shops or online; alternatively, use firm grated mozzarella)
- 4-8 tbsp ready-made tomato salsa
- 2 handfuls crisp lettuce such as Iceberg or Romaine lettuce, shredded

Method

1. For the chicken, heat a frying pan over a high heat. When the pan is hot, add the chipotle and habanero chillies and dry-fry, turning regularly, until the skins are almost completely blackened and blistered all over. Transfer the chillies to a bowl and cover them with warm water (from a kettle). Set aside to soak for 15-20 minutes, or until soft.

2. When the chillies are soft, carefully drain away the water and remove the stalks, seeds and skins using your fingers. (CAUTION: Wash your hands thoroughly after skinning and de-seeding the chillies, and don't touch your eyes during the process.) Roughly chop the chilli flesh, then transfer it to a

pestle and mortar and add the salt and olive oil. Pound the chillies to a smooth paste.

3. Stir the orange juice, oregano and garlic into the chilli paste until well combined.

4. Lay the spatchcocked chicken out onto a clean work surface. Spread the chilli marinade all over it. Set aside to marinate for at least 30 minutes, or preferably overnight (covered and chilled).

5. Meanwhile, for the frijoles, melt the butter in a large saucepan over a high heat. When the butter is foaming, add the onion and garlic and fry for 6-8 minutes, or until softened but not coloured.

6. Add the chopped coriander stalks to the mixture and continue to fry for a further 3-4 minutes, stirring well.

7. Stir the black beans and all of the tin contents (see tip) into the mixture. Bring the mixture to the boil, then reduce the heat until the mixture is simmering and simmer for 12-15 minutes, stirring regularly, until the beans are very soft and the sauce has thickened. (Garnish with the coriander leaves and chopped chilli just before serving.)

8. When the chicken has marinated, heat a large, heavy-based griddle pan or frying pan over a medium to high heat. When the pan is hot, add the marinated chicken, skin-side down.

9. Wrap a brick in aluminium foil (see tip). Place the brick on top of the chicken and continue to griddle, without moving or turning it, for 20-25 minutes, or until the chicken is completely cooked through (the chicken is cooked through if the juices run clear when a skewer is inserted into the thickest part of the meat and no trace of pink remains).

10. Remove the brick(s) from the chicken, remove the chicken from the pan and set aside to rest before carving into slices.

11. To serve, divide the chicken, frijoles, cheese, tomato salsa and lettuce e q ually among the tacos, or let people make their own tacos.

Chicken tikka and naan bread

Ingredients
For the chicken tikka
- 800g/1lb 12 oz boneless chicken legs or breasts
- 150g/5½oz yoghurt
- 50g/1¾oz unsalted butter

- 80g/2¾oz chopped fresh ginger
- ½ tsp ground cumin
- ½ tsp ground coriander
- ½ tsp red chilli powder, plus extra if re q uired
- ¼ tsp turmeric
- 2 limes, juice only
- 2 tbsp tomato purée
- ½ tsp garam masala powder
- 50ml/2fl oz oil
- salt and white pepper, to taste

For the naan bread
- 100g/3½oz plain Greek style or live yogurt, at room temperature
- 160ml/5½fl oz milk, at room temperature
- 1–2 tsp salt
- 1–2 tsp sugar
- 500g/1lb 2oz plain white flour (preferably stone-ground organic), sifted
- 1 heaped tsp baking powder
- 3 tbsp extra-virgin rapeseed oil, plus extra for kneading
- 1 heaped tbsp butter
- Nigella seeds and poppy seeds, to scatter (optional)
- 2 tbsp fresh coriander, chopped

For the salad
- 1 red onion, finely sliced
- 2 tbsp fresh coriander, chopped
- 2 tbsp fresh mint leaves, chopped

Method
1. For the chicken tikka cut the chicken into cubes large enough to be skewered (about 4cm/1½in cubes). Rub salt and pepper into the chicken and set aside.
2. In a blender, add half the yoghurt and all the remaining tikka ingredients. Blend to a smooth paste. Transfer to a large bowl and whisk in the remaining yoghurt. Taste to check for spiciness and add more chilli if preferred.
3. Mix the chicken in the yoghurt mixture. Cover with cling film and, if possible, leave the chicken to marinate in the fridge overnight, or at least 4–5 hours.

4. For the naan bread, combine the yoghurt, milk, salt and sugar with 200ml/7fl oz water. Sift the flour and baking powder into a large mixing bowl and make a well in the centre. Pour in the li q uid and 2 tablespoons of rapeseed oil. Mix to form a soft dough. Knead for 5–6 minutes, or until the dough stops looking ragged and becomes smooth. Cover the bowl with a damp tea towel and set aside to prove for 30–40 minutes. Remove the dough and knead for another minute or two, then return to the bowl. Cover and leave in a warm place for 1–2 hours.

5. For the salad, combine all the ingredients in a bowl. Refrigerate until ready to serve.

6. To cook the chicken, either preheat a grill to medium-high or prepare a barbecue. (If there is no other option you can use an oven set to its highest temperature.) Thread the chicken pieces onto metal skewers.

7. Grill the chicken for 8–10 minutes, basting occasionally with the yoghurt marinade. To check the chicken is cooked through, take one of the largest pieces and cut in half. If there is no sign of pink and the juices run clear the chicken is cooked.

8. To cook the naans, lightly oil a work surface and divide the dough into 4–6 balls. Using your fingers or an oiled rolling pin, flatten each ball into a round shape about 1cm/½in thick. Keep the remaining balls of dough under the damp tea towel as you work.

9. Heat a large, dry frying pan with a tightly-fitting lid over a medium heat. Transfer one circle of dough to the pan and cover securely with the lid. Cook the naan for 3–4 minutes. When it is golden-brown, mottled and puffed up, flip it over and cook the other side for 3–4 minutes. Repeat with the remaining dough.

10. While the naan breads are cooking, melt the butter and mix with the remaining rapeseed oil. As soon as the naans are cooked, spread them generously with the melted butter mixture and scatter with sea salt, nigella seeds and poppy seeds. Set aside for a few minutes.

11. Alternatively, preheat your oven to 250C/230C Fan/Gas 9. Place an uncooked naan on a large baking tray and bake on the top shelf one at a time. Turn when you see the bread rise and puffed. Once browned on both sides, apply the butter mixture as above.

12. To serve, scatter the naans with chopped coriander and serve with the chicken tikka and salad.

Thai roast chicken with sesame noodles and pakchoi

Ingredients
For the Thai roast chicken
• 2 red chillies, halved, seeds removed
• 150g/5¼oz creamed coconut
• 4 limes, zest and juice of 2 limes, remaining 2 limes sliced
• Handful fresh coriander
• 1 x 1.5kg/3lbs 5oz whole chicken, preferably free-range

For the sesame noodles
• 350g/12½oz fresh egg noodles
• 1 tbsp sesame seeds, toasted
• 1 tbsp sesame oil
• 2 spring onions, sliced

For the garlic pakchoi
• 1 tbsp vegetable oil
• 2 garlic cloves, crushed
• pinch sugar
• 4 heads pakchoi, halved, cores removed
• 570ml/1 pint chicken stock
• 2 tsp Thai fish sauce (nampla)
• 4 sprigs fresh coriander, to garnish

Method
1. For the Thai roast chicken, preheat the oven to 190C/350F/Gas 5.
2. Blend the chillies, creamed coconut, lime zest, lime juice and coriander in a food processor to a smooth paste.
3. Carefully push some of the paste between the skin and flesh of the chicken breasts, making sure it is evenly distributed.
4. Score the chicken thighs twice with a sharp knife right down to the bone. Carefully rub the remaining paste into the cuts and all over the chicken thighs.
5. Lay the lime slices on the bottom of a roasting tray and sit the chicken on top. Cover with aluminium foil and roast in the oven for 40 minutes. Remove

the aluminium foil, baste the chicken with any juices that have collected in the bottom of the tray and return to the oven for a further 30-40 minutes, basting occasionally, or until the chicken is cooked through.

6. Remove the chicken from the oven and set aside to rest in a warm place for five minutes.

7. Meanwhile, for the sesame noodles, cook the noodles according to the packet instructions. Drain well.

8. Mix the cooked noodles, sesame seeds, sesame oil and spring onions together in a bowl. Set aside.

9. For the garlic pakchoi, heat the oil in a frying pan over a medium heat. Fry the garlic and sugar for one minute, until the sugar has caramelised. Add the pakchoi, cut-sides down, then pour in the chicken stock and fish sauce and bring the mixture to the boil. Reduce the heat until the mixture is simmering, then cover the pan with a circle of greaseproof paper (a cartouche) and simmer for 3-4 minutes, or until the pakchoi is tender.

10. To serve, carve the chicken. Place one pakchoi half into each of four serving bowls. Twist portions of the noodles around a fork and place them in the middle of the serving bowls. Top with the some of the chicken and the remaining pakchoi halves, then drizzle with any juices from the roasting tray. Garnish with the coriander sprigs.

Roast spatchcock chicken with a burrata and slow roasted tomato salad

Ingredients
For the spatchcock chicken
- 1 x 2kg/2lb 4oz free-range chicken
- 2 red onions, q uartered
- 2 tbsp Dijon mustard
- 50g/1¾oz unsalted butter
- 2 tbsp vegetable oil
- 1 onion, finely chopped
- 2 tbsp chopped sage
- 1 lemon, zest and juice
- 50g/1¾oz dried onion flakes

For burrata and slow roasted tomato salad
• 6 plum tomatoes, halved lengthways
• 2 sprigs thyme
• Salt and freshly ground black pepper
• 3 tbsp olive oil
• 200g/7oz ciabatta, torn into small pieces
• 1 large banana shallot, finely chopped
• 2 tbsp red wine vinegar
• 6 tbsp extra virgin olive oil
• 4 tbsp capers, drained and rinsed
• 175g/6oz wood-roasted piquillo peppers, chopped (available from some supermarkets and delicatessens)
• 2 x 200g/7oz burrata mozzarella cheese, torn into pieces
• 2 handfuls basil, leaves only

Method
1. Preheat the oven to 200C/400F/Gas 6.
2. For the spatchcock chicken, place the chicken, breast-side down, onto a chopping board. Using strong kitchen scissors cut through the flesh and bone along both sides of the backbone from the tail end to the head end and completely remove the backbone. Place the chicken, breast-side down, onto a roasting tray and press it down as flat as possible. Once the chicken is flattened out, place the red onions at the bottom of the roasting tray. Turn the chicken breast-side up in the roasting tray.
3. Spread the Dijon mustard over the chicken and dot with the butter all over.
4. Heat a medium frying pan and once hot add the oil. Add the onion and cook for a couple of minutes, then add the sage, lemon zest and juice and cook for a further minute. Remove from the heat and stir in the dried onion flakes.
5. Pour the onion mix over the chicken and roast the chicken for 40-45 minutes, or until crisp, golden-brown and cooked through. (The chicken is cooked through when the juices run clear when a skewer is inserted into the thickest part of the chicken.) Remove the spatchcock chicken from the oven and rest for 5-10 minutes before serving.
6. For the slow-roasted tomatoes, preheat the oven to 150C/300F/Gas 1.
7. Place the tomatoes, cut-side up, onto a roasting tray.
8. Sprinkle with the thyme, salt and freshly ground black pepper, to taste, and

olive oil.

9. Place in the oven and cook for 1-2 hours until the moisture has mainly evaporated and the tomatoes have dried out.

10. Remove the tomatoes from the oven and leave to cool.

11. Increase the oven temperature to 220C/450F/Gas 8.

12. Place the ciabatta pieces onto a baking sheet and drizzle over two tablespoons of the olive oil. Season, to taste, with salt and freshly ground black pepper.

13. Cook in the oven for 5-7 minutes, or until crisp and golden-brown.

14. Heat the remaining tablespoon of oil in a frying pan over a medium heat. Add the shallot and fry for 2-3 minutes, or until softened.

15. Blend two-thirds of the roasted tomatoes with the red wine vinegar and the extra virgin olive oil in a food processor to a fine purée.

16. In a bowl, add half of the purée mixture to the crisp ciabatta croutons and set aside to soak for five minutes.

17. Into the other half of the purée, stir in the remaining roasted tomatoes, fried shallots, capers, pi q uillo peppers, cheese and basil leaves. Set aside.

18. To serve, carve the chicken into pieces and divide among 4-6 plates. Place the salad on the side.

Buttermilk chicken

Ingredients
- 3 garlic cloves, peeled
- 284–300ml/approx. ½ pint buttermilk
- 10g/ ⅓ oz fresh flatleaf parsley (optional)
- 1 tbsp chopped fresh rosemary or 2 tsp dried rosemary
- 1 tbsp soft light brown sugar or runny honey
- 1 tsp flaked sea salt or ½ tsp fine salt
- 1 tsp coarsely ground black pepper
- 4 chicken thighs
- 4 chicken drumsticks

Method

1. Flatten the garlic cloves with the end of a rolling pin, the side of a knife, or in a pestle and mortar. (If you chop or fully crush the garlic it could burn when the chicken is baked.) Put in a large bowl and add the buttermilk.

2. Roughly chop the leaves from half the parsley, if using, and return the rest to the fridge.

3. Stir the chopped parsley, rosemary, sugar, salt and pepper into the buttermilk. Add the chicken and turn to coat in the marinade. Cover the bowl and leave in the fridge for at least 8 hours, or overnight.

4. Preheat the oven to 200C/180C Fan/Gas 6. Line a large baking tray with foil and place a rack on top. Take the chicken out of the marinade, gently shaking off excess buttermilk and garlic. Place on the rack, with the thighs skin-side up. Discard the marinade.

5. Roast the chicken for 35–40 minutes, or until lightly browned in places and cooked through. The chicken is cooked when the juices run clear when pierced with a skewer in the thickest part. Chop the remaining parsley leaves and sprinkle over the chicken just before serving. Eat hot or cold with salad and baked potatoes, boiled new potatoes or chips.

Chicken with cheese, prosciutto and roasted courgettes

Ingredients
For the chicken
- 1 skinless chicken breast, cut in half lengthways
- 2 slices fontina cheese, the same length as the chicken breast
- 2 slices prosciutto ham, the same length as the chicken breast
- 2 sprigs fresh rosemary, same length as the chicken breast
- Plain flour, for dusting
- 10g/½oz butter
- 2 tbsp olive oil
- salt and freshly ground black pepper
- ¼ glass white wine

For the courgettes
- 3 tbsp extra virgin olive oil
- 2 courgettes, cut into rounds
- 2 tomatoes, sliced
- 2 sprigs fresh marjoram, leaves picked
- 2 tbsp grated parmesan
- Salt and freshly ground black pepper

Method

1. Preheat oven to 230C/445F/Gas 8.

2. For the chicken removes the needles from the rosemary and chop finely. Take the bare woody rosemary stem and sharpen the thickest point to create a skewer.

3. Flatten the chicken halves slightly with a meat mallet or rolling pin, then season with salt and freshly ground black pepper and sprinkle with the chopped rosemary needles.

4. Place one slice of fontina on top of each chicken piece, followed by the prosciutto.

5. Secure the stack with the rosemary branch as you would with a skewer or wooden toothpick.

6. For the courgettes drizzle one tablespoon of the olive oil into a small ovenproof dish.

7. Arrange alternate slices of tomato and courgette overlapping each other in the dish and season with salt and freshly ground black pepper.

8. Drizzle with another one tablespoon olive oil, sprinkle with the marjoram leaves and top with parmesan.

9. Place into the oven to bake for 4-5 minutes, until the cheese begins to melt and turn golden.

10. Meanwhile, dredge the bare side of the chicken with plain flour and shake off any excess.

11. Heat the butter and olive oil in a frying pan over a medium heat. When the butter is foaming add the chicken, flesh-side down first and cook on a medium heat for about two minutes, or until golden-brown, then turn the breast over and cook for one minute on the prosciutto side, until golden.

12. Turn the chicken breast over again and add the wine to the pan. Heat to boil and reduce the li q uid until almost entirely evaporated. Check the chicken breast is completely cooked through, then remove the chicken and place on a plate to rest.

13. Add a small knob of butter to the pan and melt to thicken the sauce.

14. Remove the courgettes and tomatoes from the oven and drizzle with the remaining tablespoon of the olive oil before serving.

15. Pour the sauce over the rested chicken and serve immediately with baked courgette and tomato.

Classic chicken Kiev with spring vegetables

Ingredients
- 225g/8oz unsalted butter, softened
- 1 garlic bulb, cloves peeled and crushed
- 4 tbsp chopped fresh flatleaf parsley leaves
- Vegetable oil, for deep-frying
- 4 skinless chicken breasts, wing bone left in (ask your butcher to do this for you)
- 75g/2¾oz plain flour
- 3 free-range eggs, lightly beaten
- 90g/3¼oz Japanese panko breadcrumbs
- 125g/4½oz runner beans, trimmed, cut into 4cm/1½in pieces
- 125g/4½oz fresh or frozen peas
- 4 spring onions, trimmed, white part roughly chopped
- 125g/4½oz broad beans, double podded
- 6 blanched garlic scapes (the long stalks from fresh garlic), cut into 4cm/1½in pieces (optional)
- Salt and freshly ground black pepper

Method
1. In a bowl, mix together 175g/6oz of the butter, all but one clove of garlic and half of the parsley. Season, to taste, with salt and freshly ground black pepper.
2. Place a sheet of cling film on a clean work surface. Spoon the garlic butter onto the cling film, then pull the edge of the cling film on top of the butter and mould the butter into a log shape. Twist the ends of the cling film to seal and chill in the fridge for at least an hour, or until needed.
3. Heat the oil in a deep-fat fryer to 160C. Alternatively, heat the oil in a deep, heavy-based saucepan until a breadcrumb sizzles and turns golden-brown when dropped into it. (Caution: Hot oil can be dangerous. Do not leave unattended.)
4. While the oil is heating, carefully cut a deep pocket in each of the chicken breasts, inserting the knife into the bone end, just under the bone.
5. Remove the cling film from the chilled garlic butter and slice it into 1cm/½in slices. Stuff each chicken breast with a few slices of garlic butter, pushing them into the chicken as far as possible.

6. Sprinkle the flour onto a plate. Beat the eggs in a bowl. Scatter the breadcrumbs onto another plate. Dust each chicken breast first in the flour, then dip into the beaten egg, then roll in the breadcrumbs until completely coated.

7. Carefully lower the chicken Kievs into the hot oil, two at a time, and fry for 8-10 minutes, or until the breadcrumbs are golden-brown and the chicken is cooked through. (To check that the chicken is cooked through, remove one breast from the oil using a slotted spoon and pierce in the thickest part with a skewer; the juices should run clear. Take care not to pierce the chicken too deeply in case the melted butter escapes!) Set the chicken Kievs aside on a plate lined with kitchen paper to drain and keep warm. Repeat the process with the remaining two chicken Kievs.

8. Meanwhile, place the runner beans, peas, spring onions, broad beans, the remaining clove of garlic and 25g/1oz of the remaining butter in a small saucepan. Cover with 275ml/½ pint water and bring to the boil. Reduce the heat until the water is simmering, then simmer for 3-4 minutes, or until the vegetables are tender. Drain well and return the vegetables to the pan.

9. Add the remaining 25g/1oz of butter, the remaining parsley and the garlic scapes, if using, to the pan and heat through until the butter has melted. Season, to taste, with salt and freshly ground black pepper.

10. To serve, spoon the spring vegetables into the centre of four serving plates. Top each portion with a chicken Kiev.

Cumin and yoghurt chicken with cucumber and dill salad

Ingredients
For the marinade
- 300ml/11fl oz natural yoghurt
- 2 tbsp mint or coriander, finely chopped
- 1 lemon, juice only
- 1 tbsp cumin seeds, ground
- 2 tbsp olive oil
- 2 cloves garlic, finely grated or crushed
- good pinch of pepper

For the chicken

• 1kg/2lb 2oz chicken, preferably organic, spatchcocked
• drizzle of olive oil

For the cucumber salad
• 1 large or 2 medium cucumbers
• ½ lemon, juice only
• 4 tbsp extra virgin olive oil
• 2 large tbsp chopped dill (mint or coriander is also great)
• Sea salt and freshly ground black pepper

Method
1. For the chicken, mix all the marinade ingredients together in a bowl.
2. With a sharp knife, carefully slash the chicken legs two or three times down to the bone. Rub the marinade into the chicken, massaging into the meat.
3. Place on a plate in the fridge for at least 30 minutes, but you can leave it for 4-6 hours.
4. Preheat the oven to 200C/400F/Gas 6.
5. Heat a griddle pan until very hot. Remove the chicken from the marinade, letting the excess drip off, but do not wipe clean. Pour a little olive oil onto the griddle pan then add the chicken, skin side down. Cook for 2-3 minutes on each side, until golden and scored with brown griddle marks.
6. Transfer to a roasting tin and place in the oven for 25-30 minutes, or until completely cooked through. Test the chicken is cooked by pushing a skewer into the thigh meat - if the juices run clear the chicken is cooked.
7. Remove from the oven and leave to rest for 5-10 minutes.
8. For the cucumber salad, cut the cucumbers into halves lengthways and scoop out the watery seeds.
9. Cut the cucumber into wedges and place in a bowl. Add the remaining ingredients and toss together to coat. Season to taste with more lemon juice or salt and freshly ground black pepper.
10. To serve, carve the chicken into eight pieces (legs, thighs and breasts). Place the cucumber salad into a pile on a plate and a bit of chicken alongside. Serve with crusty bread or a couscous salad.

Pulled chicken with barbecue sauce and baked

potatoes

Ingredients
For the pulled chicken
- 1 tsp smoked paprika
- 1 tsp freshly ground black pepper
- ½ tsp salt
- 4 chicken legs
- 4 x 300g/10½oz floury potatoes, such as King Edward or Maris Piper

For the barbecue sauce
- 6 tbsp tomato ketchup
- 3 tbsp clear honey
- 1½ tbsp Worcestershire sauce

For the sweetcorn
- 4 frozen mini corn-on-the-cobs
- 25g/1oz butter
- Salt and freshly ground black pepper

To serve
- Handful chopped fresh flatleaf parsley or chives (optional)
- 4 tbsp soured cream and chive dip, or reduced-fat crème fraîche (optional)

Method
1. Preheat the oven to 180C/160C Fan/Gas 4. Line the base and sides of a baking tray with aluminium foil.

2. In a bowl, mix together the paprika, black pepper and salt until well combined.

3. Put the chicken legs on a chopping board and carefully score the skin of each leg 5-6 times using a sharp knife.

4. Roll the scored skin of each chicken leg in the salt and paprika mixture, pressing down to coat evenly. Place the spiced chicken legs on the prepared baking tray.

5. Wash and pat dry the potatoes and prick each 3-4 times with a fork to stop the skins splitting when they are baked. Add the potatoes to the baking tray. Bake the chicken and potatoes in the oven for 1 hour.

6. Meanwhile, for the barbecue sauce, in a bowl, mix together all of the barbecue sauce ingredients until well combined.

7. Remove the chicken from the oven and increase the oven temperature to 220C/200C Fan/Gas 7.

8. Brush the chicken legs all over with the barbecue sauce, then return the chicken and potatoes to the oven and continue to cook for a further 12-15 minutes, or until the potatoes are tender and the chicken is cooked through with sticky, dark-brown skin. (The chicken is cooked through if the juices run clear when the meat is pierced with a skewer in the thickest part, and no trace of pink remains.)

9. Meanwhile, for the sweetcorn, half-fill a saucepan with water and bring it to the boil. Add the frozen corn-on-the-cobs and return the water to the boil, then cook the sweetcorn according to the packet instructions, until tender. Drain well, then return to the saucepan and stir in the butter until melted. Season well with salt and freshly ground black pepper. (Alternatively, cook in the microwave according to the packet instructions, then add the butter and seasoning.)

10. Just before serving, shred the chicken meat using two forks to pull the meat apart. Discard the bones, but keep the skin (thinly slice it with a sharp knife if you cannot shred it).

11. Serve the pulled barbecue chicken with the buttered corn-on-the-cobs and the baked potatoes alongside. Sprinkle over the parsley or chives. Serve the soured cream and chive dip (or crème fraîche) in dipping bowls alongside, if using.

Kale and q uinoa salad with orange tahini dressing

Ingredients
For the kale and quinoa sauté
- 350g/12oz q uinoa
- 1 tbsp extra virgin olive oil
- 2 tsp coconut oil
- 600g/1lb 5½oz kale, tough stalks discarded, leaves shredded, washed
- 1 fat garlic clove, finely chopped
- 1 large handful chopped fresh coriander or flatleaf parsley, to garnish
- 1 unwaxed orange, zest only, finely sliced

For the tahini dressing
- 2½ tbsp tahini
- 2 tbsp extra virgin olive oil

- 1 garlic clove
- 6 tbsp warm (boiled) water
- 4 tbsp orange juice
- Freshly ground black pepper

Method

1. put the quinoa in a bowl and cover with approximately 700ml/1¼ pints cold water. Set aside to soak overnight (or for at least 8 hours).

2. Drain the q uinoa and transfer to a very large saucepan. Cover with 350ml/12fl oz water and bring to the boil. Reduce the heat and simmer for 10-12 minutes, or until the quinoa is tender.

3. Drain the q uinoa and put in a large mixing bowl. Drizzle over the olive oil and season with sea salt.

4. Meanwhile, for the dressing, whisk together all of the dressing ingredients until smooth, creamy and well combined, adding a splash of warm water to loosen the mixture if necessary. Season with pepper. Set aside.

5. Heat the coconut oil in a frying pan over a medium heat until melted. Add the kale and stir-fry for 1-2 minutes, adding the garlic after 1 minute. Continue to fry until the kale is just tender, then tip it into the q uinoa and stir to combine.

6. To serve, divide the kale and quinoa sauté equally among 4 plates, garnish with the orange zest. Drizzle over the tahini dressing and scatter over the herbs.

Peanut and dried mango-crusted partridge with curry leaf and tomato quinoa

Ingredients

- 4 partridges, cut in half lengthways
- 1 tsp salt
- 2 tbsp malt vinegar
- 2 tbsp ginger and garlic paste (made by blending a 1cm/½in piece of ginger and 1 garlic clove together with 1 tsp of water)
- 1 tsp cumin seeds
- 200ml/7fl oz Greek yoghurt
- 2 tsp dried mango powder
- 3 tbsp roasted unsalted peanuts, coarsely crushed

• 2 fresh hot green chillies, finely chopped
• 1 tbsp vegetable oil
• 2 tbsp coriander stems, finely chopped
• ½ lemon, juice only
• 4 wooden skewers, soaked in warm water

For the quinoa
• 150g/5oz quinoa
• 3 tbsp vegetable or corn oil
• 1 dried red chilli, broken into 3 pieces
• 1 tsp mustard seeds
• 20 fresh curry leaves
• 1 large onion, finely chopped
• 1 green chilli, finely chopped
• 1cm/½-inch piece fresh root ginger, finely chopped
• 2 tomatoes, coarsely chopped
• 1½ tsp salt
• 1 tsp red chilli powder
• ½ tsp sugar
• 1 tbsp fresh coriander or basil, finely chopped
• ½ lemon, juice only

Method
1. For the partridge, preheat the oven to 200C/290F/Gas 6 and preheat the grill to high.
2. Place the partridge in a non-reactive dish. Whisk the salt, malt vinegar and ginger and garlic paste together in a small bowl.
3. Spoon the paste over the partridge and leave to marinate for a few minutes.
4. Meanwhile, heat a frying pan until hot, add the cumin seeds and lightly fry until fragrant.
5. Tip the cumin seeds into a pestle and mortar and lightly crush them, then place in a bowl with the yoghurt, dried mango, crushed roasted peanuts, chopped green chillies and oil and whisk together.
6. Add the coriander stems and lemon juice, then spread this mixture over the partridge. If you have time, you can leave the partridge to marinate for at least 30 minutes.

7. Thread the partridge onto the soaked wooden skewers, place on a roasting tray and transfer to the oven to cook for 8-10 minutes. Remove and then place under the grill to cook for a further three minutes, or until cooked to your liking. Remove the meat from the skewers and leave in a warm place to rest.

8. For the q uinoa, soak the q uinoa in cold water for 15 minutes, then drain and rinse.

9. Place the q uinoa in a saucepan with 300ml/10fl oz of salted water, bring to the boil then reduce the heat and simmer for about 15 minutes, or until the grains are cooked, but still retain some bite - q uinoa develops a white ring round the circumference of each grain when it is nearly ready. Drain off any excess water.

10. Heat the oil in a heavy-based pan and add the red chilli and mustard seeds. (CAUTION: keep the pan well away from the eyes and face as the mustard seeds may pop.) Allow the seeds to crackle and splutter for about 30 seconds, then add the curry leaves.

11. When the curry leaves are crisp, add the onion and cook for 3-4 minutes, until starting to turn golden-brown. Add the green chilli and ginger and stir for one minute.

12. Add the tomato, salt and chilli powder and cook over a medium heat for 3-4 minutes, until most of the moisture from the tomato has evaporated.

13. Add the cooked quinoa into the pan and mix for 1-2 minutes, until heated through. Add the sugar, coriander or basil and lemon juice and stir to combine.

14. To serve, spoon the q uinoa into the centre of each of four serving plates. Top each serving of q uinoa with two halves of partridge.

Quinoa and halloumi burger

Ingredients
- 250g/9oz q uinoa
- 250ml/9fl oz vegetable stock or water
- 2 free-range eggs, beaten
- 3 tbsp gram flour
- 3 tsp dried oregano or thyme
- ½ tsp chilli flakes (or chopped fresh chilli, to taste)
- 3 garlic cloves, crushed

• 5 spring onions, trimmed and finely sliced
• 225g/8oz halloumi, diced
• 1 tbsp ghee, for frying
• Salt and freshly ground black pepper

Method
1. Put the q uinoa in a bowl and cover with approximately 500ml/18fl oz cold water. Add a pinch of salt. Set aside to soak overnight (or for at least 8 hours). Drain well.
2. Bring the stock to the boil in a large saucepan. Add the quinoa, stir once, then simmer for 10-12 minutes, or until tender. Remove from the heat and drain well. Set aside to cool.
3. Preheat the oven to 190C/170C Fan/Gas 5.
4. In a large mixing bowl, beat together the eggs, gram flour, herbs, chilli, and garlic until smooth and well combined. Stir in the spring onions, halloumi and quinoa. Season with salt and pepper. Add a little more gram flour or water if needed.
5. Shape the burger mixture into 16 e q ual-shaped patties in your hands.
6. Heat the ghee in a large frying pan over a medium-high heat. When the fat is smoking, add the burger patties, shape with a spoon in the pan. You may need to do this in batches. Fry for 3-4 minutes, or until a golden-brown crust forms, then gently flip with a spatula and fry the other side.
7. Transfer the fried burgers to a roasting tray. When all of the burgers have been fried, cook them in the oven for a further 12-15 minutes, or until cooked through.
8. Serve with a green salad with red onion and avocado.

Cornish ling, grapefruit and prawn dressing, spiced quinoa and lemon yoghurt

Ingredients
For the q uinoa
• 50g/1¾oz q uinoa
• 3 tbsp olive oil
• 1 tsp salt
• ½ tsp dill seeds
• ½ tsp fennel seed

- ¼ tsp cumin seed
- ¼ tsp ground cinnamon
- 1 tsp flat leaf parsley, finely chopped
- 1 tsp dill, finely chopped
- 1 tsp chives, finely chopped
- Salt and freshly ground black pepper
- 150g/5½oz winter salad leaves
- 1 tbsp balsamic vinegar

For the ling
- 4 x 125g/4½oz Cornish ling pieces, skinned
- Salt, to taste
- 2 tbsp olive oil
- Lemon juice, to taste
- 115g/4oz Greek-style yoghurt

For the grapefruit dressing
- 50ml/2fl oz grapefruit juice
- 50ml/2fl oz olive oil
- Pinch salt
- 50g/2oz peeled cooked prawns
- 1 tbspflatleaf parsley
- 10g/½oz capers

Method
1. For the q uinoa, place all but about a teaspoon of the quinoa into a saucepan with 200ml/7fl oz water, one tablespoon of the olive oil and the salt and bring to the boil. Reduce the heat and simmer for 10 minutes then cover with cling film and allow to steam in a warm place until the quinoa has cooled. Place the cooled q uinoa in a large mixing bowl.

2. Heat a frying pan until medium hot, add one tablespoon of the oil, the reserved q uinoa, dill seed, fennel seed, cumin seed and ground cinnamon and toast for one minute.

3. Pour the mixture onto the cooked quinoa then stir in the herbs. Mix well and season to taste with salt and freshly ground black pepper.

4. Toss the winter leaves with a little of the q uinoa, the balsamic vinegar and the last of the olive oil.

5. For the ling, preheat the oven to 180C/350F/Gas 4. Season the ling well

with salt.
6. Heat a non-stick frying pan until hot, add the olive oil. Add the ling and cook on each side until lightly golden-brown.
7. Remove the ling from the pan, and place onto a baking tray. Bake in the oven for 3-4 minutes.
8. Remove the baking tray from the oven and season the ling with a little salt and lemon juice.
9. Place the yoghurt into a bowl and season, to taste, with lemon juice and salt. Mix well.
10. For the grapefruit and prawn dressing, place the grapefruit juice, olive oil, 25ml/1fl oz water and salt into a jug and stir until the salt dissolves. Pour the dressing into a small saucepan and heat through, then add the prawns, parsley and capers.
11. To serve, spoon lemon yoghurt around 4 plates, and place a pile of q uinoa in the centre of each plate. Top with a piece of ling, and spoon the grapefruit and prawn dressing over the top. Serve the salad leaves alongside.

Spiced monkfish tail with pickled beetroot and lemon, herby q uinoa

Ingredients
For the spiced monkfish tail
- 1 monkfish tail, trimmed
- 2 tsp medium curry powder
- 2 tbsp ground cumin
- 4 tbsp olive oil
- Salt and freshly ground black pepper

For the pickled beetroot
- 2 tbsp olive oil
- 2 banana shallots, chopped
- 4 cooked beetroot, peeled and diced
- ½ tsp garam masala
- ½ tsp black onion seeds
- pinch dried chilli flakes
- 2 tbsp red wine vinegar
- 2 tbsp caster sugar

For the q uinoa
• 200g/7oz q uinoa
• 400ml/14fl oz chicken stock
• 1 lemon, zest and juice
• Selection of soft herbs, such as chervil, parsley and coriander
• olive oil, to taste
To garnish
• Salad leaves

Method
1. For the monkfish tail, preheat the oven to 200C/180C Fan/Gas 6.
2. Season the monkfish with the curry powder, cumin, salt and pepper. Heat a large frying pan and add the oil. Once hot add the monkfish tail and cook on all sides until golden-brown. Place in the oven for 6-8 minutes, then set aside to rest.
3. For the beetroot, heat a sauté pan and add the oil. Once hot add the shallots and cook for 2-3 minutes. Add the beetroot and spices and cook for 2-3 minutes. Add the vinegar and sugar and cook for 5 minutes.
4. For the q uinoa, cook the q uinoa in a saucepan using the chicken stock according to the packet instructions. Remove and allow to cool before adding the lemon juice and zest and chopped herbs. Dress with the olive oil.
5. To serve, dot the q uinoa and pickled beetroot around the plate. Cut the monkfish tail into pieces and place on top of the q uinoa. Garnish with the salad leaves.

BOTTOM LINE

Individuals with MS are at higher risk for emotional disorders, which can significantly disrupt family, work, and social life. These mood disorders are highly treatable through a combination of psychiatric and psychological therapy and medication treatment.

The resources exist, but the delivery of these treatments is not always well-implemented. Learning to address your concerns about your emotional reactions with your MS neurologist and other members of your healthcare team is essential. People with MS must not only focus on the physical symptoms of MS, but also on the emotional and psychological symptoms.

When needed, ask your physician and/or nurse to refer you to mental-health professionals who are skilled in this area and who ideally have experience with MS or other chronic conditions.

Please note, however, that mental-health professionals who specialize in MS are extremely limited. According to MSAA's client services department, "When people call for a referral, we refer them first to their MS center or neurologist, who may have someone to recommend. As a second option, we advise people with insurance to check with their provider for mental-health professionals who have a specialty in chronic illness, pain management, or neurological disorders. We explain that not every therapist may be a good match for every person, and that individuals may need to schedule a few introductory sessions with different providers before finding someone they are comfortable with."

We hope that this article will help individuals with MS who are experiencing emotional or psychological issues to know that they are not alone – and that they should not feel embarrassed over these symptoms that they cannot control. Seeking help by discussing these issues with your doctor is the first step toward returning to a happier and more satisfying q uality of life.